42 Cardio Workouts and Other Ideas To Make Exercise Fun and Not Boring

Kelli Rae

42 Cardio Workouts and Other Ideas To Make Exercise Fun and Not Boring

All rights reserved
Copyright ©2015 Active Passion Publications, LLC

The information provided in this book is designed to provide helpful information on the subjects discussed. This book is not meant to be used, nor should it be used, to diagnose or treat any medical condition. For diagnosis or treatment of any medical problem, consult your own physician. The publisher and author are not responsible for any specific health or allergy needs that may require medical supervision and are not liable for any damages or negative consequences from any treatment, action, application or preparation, to any person reading or following the information in this book.

No part of this book may be reproduced or transmitted in any form or by any means, electronic or mechanical, including photocopying, recording or by any information storage and retrieval system, without the permission in writing from Active Passion Publications, LLC.

CONTENTS

Introduction	1
Part 1: Ideas	3
Part 2: Cardio Routines	8
Part 3: Other Ideas	51
Thank You!	54
You May Also Enjoy	54

Introduction

This short book is intended for people who need a little mix-up with their cardio routine at the gym. You may not enjoy cardio very much, or you may be short on time and not sure how to get a good workout. Let's face it - cardio can be INCREDIBLY BORING if you do the same thing all of the time, day after day. Your body can also get used to the same routine, making it harder and harder to reach any goals you may have.

In part one, I have included several ideas on how to mix up your cardio routine. I have used all of these tips myself, but there are certainly other routines out these besides what I have provided. Feel free to be creative! In part two, you will find specific cardio routines that you can use at the gym so you don't even need to think about what to do. You can choose routines using a variety of equipment, from the elliptical, stairs, treadmill, bike and even no equipment at all. Feel free to use your creativity and go beyond what is in this book. The possibilities are endless!

In part three, I will give you some suggestions about other things to switch up besides doing cardio on a machine. They may be small changes, but it may be just the thing that you need.

If you have any questions or comments about anything fitness related, whether it's about these routines or something else, please email me anytime at kelliraefit@gmail.com.

Part 1: Ideas

Phone Number

Choose a phone number. If you need help deciding on one, randomly choose a number from your phone. This will help force you to do something a little bit more challenging. If you choose all of the numbers, will you push yourself hard enough? There is a possibility of choosing "easier" numbers. Whatever you decide, these numbers are going to represent the change in levels or incline on the machine that you have chosen.

For example, let's pick the random number (888)280-3321 for a 20 minute session. After you are warmed up, do 2 minutes at level 8. Repeat this sequence 3 times, which will be for the first 3 numbers. Then do 2 minutes at level 2, 2 minutes at level 8 and so forth until you finish all of the numbers. If you choose a machine (such as a treadmill) where there are 2 items to change (level and incline), keep one of them at a constant yet challenging level, and change the other one. If you choose a phone number that has a zero, that represent level 10. If you wish to have your workout be shorter or longer than 20 minutes, adjust each number appropriately.

Tabatas

Tabatas are another type of interval training where

you go hard for 20 seconds and then rest for 10 seconds. You will repeat this cycle for a total of 4 minutes and then rest for 1 minute. Repeat this again for a total of 20 minutes and you will definitely get a great workout. If you are doing the workout correctly, it should be very intense and the time will pass very quickly.

The easiest way to keep track of time is on a cardio machine of your choice. If you are doing a routine off the machine, there are a few other options. My personal favorite and preferred method is to use a timer app on a smartphone. This means you can go anywhere and not have an excuse. My favorite is called Seconds Free because you will be able to track all different kinds of intervals, including tabatas. If you would like something different, search for "tabata" or "interval" on your device and there will be several free options. Another option is to find a clock at the gym that is digital. As a last resort, you could use a clock in the gym with a seconds hand. However, make sure you are able to see it clearly and able to keep up a high same intensity.

Random Intervals
You could also choose your own intervals. For example, you could go on the elliptical, do 30 seconds of intense work followed by 45 seconds of a recovery speed for a total of 20 minutes. Or you could go to the treadmill for 20 minutes. Do an intense 20 second sprint, and then do a quick paced walk for 40 seconds. Repeat. Or you could even pick any machine and make it a game for yourself. Go as

fast as you can for as long as you can. Then rest at a recovery pace for 30 seconds to a minute. Repeat. Aim to go for a specific distance or time. Do this again in a couple of weeks and try to beat your time or distance the next time you do the routine. If none of this sounds fun, use your imagination because the possibilities are endless.

If you choose this type of workout, I would recommend writing down the workout you would like to do. I suggest this because when the workout gets tough, your body may try to talk you out of a certain intensity. Do not listen! However when it's written down, it may be easier to follow because it's right there and you just have to follow it. Or you can follow one of the routines I have layed out in part two.

Pyramids
I consider this type of interval a little more advanced because you progressively do a longer amount of intensity in a short period of time. I call it a pyramid because you will start to do more intense work the longer you go in the routine.

Start with 1 minute at a low speed. Then increase your level by 8 (or an incredibly substantial amount if this isn't a challenge on your machine). Do this for 10 seconds, and then 50 seconds of your original, slow speed. Then go back up to the fast speed for 20 seconds, then 40 seconds slow. 30 seconds fast, 30 seconds slow and repeat this pattern until you do 60 seconds fast, 0 seconds slow.

If you want the workout to be even more difficult, repeat this pattern backwards (60 seconds fast, 0 slow, 50 seconds fast, 10 slow, etc).

Music Intervals

Another creative way to mix up your workouts is to use music intervals, and there are several ways you can do this. First, pick a good music station or several songs you enjoy. I think it works best to choose songs with varying tempos.

Once you're on the machine, increase or decrease your speeds depending on the tempo of the music. The song may start slow and speed up, so this is what you should do on your machine. Or, you could alternate your speeds according to the song. Go faster for one complete song, and then use the next song for recovery by going a little bit slower. Or even better, get creative and use both methods. For one song, go according to the tempo. Then for the next song, go really fast. Then for the third song, go slower and use it for recovery. Repeat.

Hopping Off Equipment

Who says you need to stay on the equipment for the entire duration? You don't - there are no rules and this is a really good way to not get bored.

There are hundreds of different options for this. One example is to pick your favorite machine in the gym. Of course, start with a warm-up and then do 5 minutes at a good pace. Then hop off and do body weight squats for a minute. Repeat this cycle for 25 minutes. If you get bored with doing squats, you could do some push-ups, mountain climbers, pop squats, jump lunges or a numerous amount of other exercises in between. It will definitely change up the pace.

Changing Equipment
Another thing you could do is change equipment. Pick your three favorite machines and do 10 minutes on each one. If you don't have a favorite, pick three at random or ask a stranger in the gym to pick. Even though you will only be on the equipment for 10 minutes at a time, make sure to keep up a good pace.

Using Weights
Another fun thing to try is cardio with weights. For safety reasons, I highly recommend sticking with the treadmill.

First, choose a pair of dumbbells and start with a light weight until you get used to doing this. From there, you have many different options. You could just hold them to the sides while you walk for extra resistance. Or, you could hold them in a static bicep curl. Or, you could even do some bicep curls. This may also be a good option if you are short on time. You could do several different upper body movements while walking and it will become a full body workout.

Part 2: Cardio Routines

Before doing any of the following routines, please make sure that you get a good warm-up. This can be as simple as 3-5 minutes walking on the treadmill at a slow, but steady pace. If you see a routine that you like under a machine that you do not have access to, please feel free to modify the routine to be appropriate for another machine.

You know your own self better than I do. You want to push yourself, but you don't want to kill yourself. These are ideas to help you as a guide, but please always check with your doctor before beginning any new exercise regimen.

Finally, when you are done with these routines, make sure to get a cool down. Please do not walk straight out of the gym immediately after finishing this routine. Doing this will not be good for your body.

Arc Trainer 1

Keep the resistance at 20 and keep a good, steady pace for the entire workout
For 3 minutes, put the incline to 6 in this order (6, 5, 4, 9, 1, 8)
1 minute, pedal backwards
3 minutes, put the incline to 5
1 minute, pedal backwards
3 minutes, incline to 4
1 minute, pedal backwards
3 minutes, incline to 9
1 minute, pedal backwards
3 minutes, incline to 1
1 minute, pedal backwards
3 minutes, incline to 8
1 minute, pedal backwards

Arc Trainer 2

Pick a random phone number
Keep the incline at 5 for entire session.
Every 3 minutes, change the resistance based on the number. You will always need to add a zero at the end.
If there is a zero in the phone number you choose, keep the same resistance as the previous number, but pedal backwards instead of forwards.
For example, for phone number 623-780-5702, start at 60, then 20, then 30, etc.

Arc Trainer 3

Start with an incline of 4 and resistance of 30
For 2 minutes, go at a good, steady pace
1 minute sprint
2 minutes, good, steady pace
1 minute sprint
Hop off and do 25 pop squats
Repeat this cycle 3 more times, increasing the incline by 1 and the resistance by 10 each time you start a new cycle

Arc Trainer 4

Keep a steady pace throughout the workout
Minute 0-3 - incline 3-6, resistance 15-30
Min 3-5:30 - incline 0-3, resistance 30-45
Min 5:30-8 - incline 0-3, resistance 15-30
Min 8-13 - Repeat minutes 3-8
Min 13-15:30 - incline 7-10, resistance 45-60
Min 15:30-18 - max incline, resistance 30-45
Min 18-23 - Repeat minutes 13-18

AMT 1

Use medium to long strides throughout, UNLESS STATED

Minute 0-2 - resistance 0

Min 2-6 - resistance 5

Min 6-8 - resistance 5-10

Min 8-9 - resistance 10-15, stepping motion

Repeat min 6-9 two more times

Finish with 5 minutes, resistance 5-10

AMT 2

Start with 5 minutes, long strides, resistance of 10
1 minute, short strides, resistance of 15
1 minute, stepping motion, resistance of 20
Repeat this cycle 4 more times

Bike 1

Keep a good, steady pace throughout the workout UNLESS it says sprint
2 minutes, level 1
2 minutes, level 10
1 minute, level 5 SPRINT
2 minutes, level 2
2 minutes, level 9
1 minute, level 6 SPRINT
2 minutes, level 3
2 minutes, level 8
1 minute, level 7 SPRINT
2 minutes, level 4
2 minutes, level 7
1 minute, level 5 SPRINT

Bike 2

Start pedaling at level 1 for one song
Sprint for 1 minute
Increase to level 2 and pedal for one song
Go to level 1 and sprint for 1 minute
Level 3 and pedal for one song
Level 2 and sprint for 1 minute
Level 4 and pedal for one song
Level 3 and sprint for 1 minute
Level 2 and pedal for one song
Level 1 and sprint for 1 minute

Bike 3

Choose a random phone number
Every 2 minutes, change the resistance based on the number. If there is a zero in the phone number you choose, make this level 10.
After you have completed the entire phone number, do the following series:
-25 squats
-25 jumping jacks
-10 push ups
-25 mountain climbers
-30 alternating lunges

Bike 4

Start at level 1 and pedal for 2 minutes
Then go to level 2 and pedal for 2 minutes
Tabata time! Machine should still be at level 2.
Sprint for 20 seconds, pedal at a slower pace for 10 seconds
Repeat this 7 more times (for a total of 4 minutes of work)
Pedal at level 1 for 1 minute
Increase to level 3
Sprint for 20 seconds, pedal at a slower pace for 10 seconds
Repeat this 7 more times (for a total of 4 minutes of work)
Pedal at level 1 for 1 minute

Bike 5

Keep all pedaling at a steady pace, but still push yourself
Start at level 2 and pedal for 3 minutes
Go to level 6 and pedal for 1 minute
Level 8 for 30 seconds
Level 10 for 30 seconds
Level 3 for 2 minutes
Level 7 for 1 minute
Level 8 for 30 seconds
Level 11 for 30 seconds
Level 2 for 3 minutes
Level 5 for 2 minutes
Level 7 for 1 minute
Level 8 for 30 seconds
Level 10 for 30 seconds
Level 2 for 2 minutes

Bike 6

Start at level 3 for 3 minutes at a steady pace
Hop off and do 50 squats
Level 4 for 3 minutes
Hop off and do 50 jumping jacks
Level 5 for 3 minutes
Hop off and do 100 calf raises
Level 6 for 3 minutes
Hop off and do 50 mountain climbers
For the next 4 minutes, keep the level at 3
Sprint for 20 minutes, pedal slower for 10 seconds
Repeat 7 more times for a total of 4 minutes
Go to level 1 and pedal for 1 minute

Elliptical 1

Begin pedaling at a moderate pace at level 3
Every 2 minutes, change from FW to BW and vice versa
Repeat this for 8 minutes
Decrease the level to 2
Sprint for 20 seconds, then go at a slower pace for 10 seconds
Repeat this 7 more times (for a total of 4 minutes of work)
Slower pace for 1 minute
Increase the level to 3
Sprint for 20 seconds, then go at a slower pace for 10 seconds
Repeat this 7 more times (for a total of 4 minutes of work)
Slower pace for 1 minute
Increase the level to 4
Sprint for 20 seconds, then go at a slower pace for 10 seconds
Repeat this 7 more times (for a total of 4 minutes of work)
Slower pace for 1 minute

Elliptical 2

Begin pedaling at a moderate pace at level 3
Maintain the moderate pace for 3 minutes
Sprint for 1 minute
Change directions and pedal backwards at a moderate pace for 1 minute
Go forwards, increase the level to 5 for 2 minutes
Sprint for 1 minute
Go backwards at a moderate pace for 1 minute
Repeat the routine two more times for a total of 27 minutes

Elliptical 3

Begin at level 1 for 1 minute at a moderate pace
Increase to level 3 for 2 minutes and increase your speed
1 minute sprint
Hop off and do 20 pop squats and 20 sumo squats
Repeat this sequence 4 times

Elliptical 4

Your choice - start at a good level for you
Pedal backwards for 1 minute at a moderate pace
Pedal forwards for 1 minute at a slightly faster pace
Double the level and sprint for 1 minute
Hop off and do 20 side to side jumps and 20 jump lunges
Repeat this sequence 4 times

Elliptical 5

(If possible) set the incline to an 8
Pick a phone number (including area code)
Every 3 minutes, change the resistance based on the phone number.
Ex: phone number you pick is 614-378-1414
Minute 5-8, resistance 6
Minute 8-11, resistance 1
Follow this pattern until all of the numbers in the phone number have been used.

Elliptical 6

Minute 0-3 - steady pace; no resistance
Min 3-6 - increase level to 3 and go at a faster, steady pace
Min 7 - 10 seconds sprint, 50 seconds steady
Min 8 - 15 seconds sprint, 45 seconds steady
Min 9 - 20 seconds sprint, 40 seconds steady
Min 10 - 25 seconds sprint, 35 seconds steady
Min 11 - 30 seconds sprint, 30 seconds steady
Min 12 - steady pace, no sprint
Increase level to 4
Min 13 - 10 seconds sprint, 50 seconds steady
Min 14 - 15 seconds sprint, 45 seconds steady
Min 15 - 20 seconds sprint, 40 seconds steady
Min 16 - 25 seconds sprint, 35 seconds steady
Min 17 - 30 seconds sprint, 30 seconds steady
Min 18-19 - steady pace, no sprint
10 minutes of abs

Stairmill 1

1 minute - Level 6
10 seconds - Level 14
50 seconds - Level 6
20 seconds - Level 14
40 seconds - Level 6
30 seconds - Level 14
30 seconds - Level 6
40 seconds - Level 14
20 seconds - Level 6
50 seconds - Level 14
10 seconds - Level 6
60 seconds - Level 14
Repeat this sequence 1 or 2 more times

Stairmill 2

Your choice - start at a moderate level for you.
Please note that depending on the machine, it could calculate the level in stairs per minute or at a certain number, such as 1-20.
Minute 0-3 - moderate pace
Min 3-6 - Increase level by 1 (or by 5 stairs per minute)
Min 6-10 - Do 4 minutes of sprints. For 30 seconds, go at a moderate level and then sprint for 30 seconds at a higher level
Min 10-16 - Step sideways, 3 minutes right side then 3 minutes left side
Min 16-20 - Do another round of sprints, just like in minutes 6-10
Min 20-24 - back to a moderate pace

Stairmaster 1

Choose a set of dumbbells and begin at level 7
Go for 2 minutes at a good pace
1 minute sprint
2 minutes at a good pace
Hop off, take your dumbbells and do the following sequence -
-20 bicep curls
-20 lunges
-20 shoulder presses
Repeat this sequence two to three more times, increasing the level by 1 at the start of each new round.

Stairmaster 2

Begin at a comfortable level and step at a good pace for 5 minutes
30 second sprint
1 minute slower pace
Increase the level by 1
30 second sprint
1 minute slower pace
Hop off and do 10 push ups
Repeat this sequence until you cannot increase the levels any more

Stairmaster 3

Begin at level 6.
Go at a good pace for 4 minutes
Flip around, stand on machine backwards and go for 1 minute.
Flip back around, increase the level by 1.
Repeat this sequence 4 times

Treadmill 1

Throughout the entire workout, take nice, long strides and squeeze your glutes.
Walk at 2.5 with an incline of 0 for 3 minutes
Increase the speed to 2.8-3.0 with an incline of 10
*DO NOT hang onto the front or sides. Make sure to keep good form, but slow down the pace if it's too fast for you.

Treadmill 2

Keep the incline at 0 for the entire workout
Walk at 3.2-3.5 for 5 minutes
Tabata time!
Sprint for 20 seconds, then hop to the sides for 10 seconds. Don't stop the speed of the treadmill
Repeat this 7 more times (for a total of 4 minutes of work)
Walk for 1 minute at 3.2-3.5
Repeat the tabatas 2 more times for a total workout of 20 minutes

Treadmill 3

I recommend some good music for this workout
Keep the incline at 2.0 for the entire workout
Walk at a medium-fast pace for one song
Jog for one song
Fast jog for one song
Walk at a medium pace for one song
For the next song, alternate between jogging and sprinting. Push yourself to your limits. Go with the flow of the music.
Walk at a medium pace for the last song

Treadmill 4

Pick a set of light to medium dumbbells.
3 minutes, hold weights to sides, walk at a medium pace, 0 incline
3 minutes, static bicep curls, walk at same pace, 3 incline
3 minutes, shoulder press, increase pace by .2, 0 incline
Hop off the treadmill and do the following:
-25 squats
-25 crunches
-25 chest press
-25 flys
Get back on the treadmill
3 minutes, hold weights to sides, walk at medium pace, 10 incline

Treadmill 5

Keep the incline at 0 for the entire workout
Minute 0-3 - walk at a steady pace
Min 3-7 - steady jog
Min 7-10 - 30 seconds sprint, 30 seconds steady jog
Min 10-14 - 15 seconds FAST and HARD sprint, 45 seconds hop to the side
Min 14-20 - steady jog

Treadmill 6

Minute 0-3 - incline 10, speed 3.4
Min 3-7:30 - incline 15, speed 3.0
Min 7:30-8 - REST (step to sides)
Min 8-11 - incline 15, speed 3.4
Min 11-11:30 - REST (step to sides)
Min 11:30-13 - incline 10, speed 4.0
Min 13-14 - REST (step to sides)
Min 14-16 - incline 10, speed 4.0
Min 16-17 - REST (step to sides)
Min 17-20 - incline 5, speed 3.5

Rowing Machine 1

Row for 500 meters at a medium, steady pace
Hop off and do 20 push ups
Row for 250 meters at a sprint
Hop off and do 50 mountain climbers
Row for 500 meters at a medium, steady pace
Hop off and do 50 fast squats
Row for 250 meters at a sprint
Hop off and do 25 pop squats

Rowing Machine 2

Row at a moderate pace for 4 minutes
Go hard for 1 minute
Hop off and do 25 pop squats
Repeat this 2 more times

Triathlon Workout

You will need an elliptical, bike, treadmill and timer. You will do ½ mile to 1 ½ miles on each machine based on your fitness level. Choose a distance that is a challenge for you. Keep the distance the same for each piece of equipment. So if you choose ½ mile, do this for the elliptical, bike and treadmill.
Time yourself from start to finish, and record time when completed.
Do this same routine in a month with the same distance and see how much you will improve.

Multiple Machines 1

Hop on the treadmill for 15 minutes at a good walking pace (3.0-3.5) at a 2.0 incline.
Hop on the elliptical for 15 minutes, maintaining at least 140 strides per minute.
Finish with 10 minutes of abs

Multiple Machines 2

Set stairmill or stairmaster on the interval program for 20 minutes. Your choice. Push yourself throughout entire program.
Go to the treadmill and jog a mile

Multiple Machines 3

Back to the basics! Keep a good pace on each machine and do -
8 minutes elliptical
8 minutes stair master
8 minutes treadmill

Multiple Machines 4

Row for 1000 meters
Jump rope 1 minute
High knee jog 1 minute
Jumping jacks 1 minute
15 burpees
Jog on the treadmill for 1 mile
Jump rope 1 minute
Mountain climbers 1 minute
15 pop squats
Elliptical for 10 minutes - keep a good pace
Jump rope 1 minute
100 squats

Multiple Machines 5

Jog for 2 miles
Stairs for 5 minutes at a good pace
Elliptical for 10 minutes, level 10
Treadmill for 10 minutes, sprinting for 30 seconds and resting for 30 seconds
Walk at a good pace for 5 minutes

Multiple Machines 6

Start on the treadmill and do the following -
4 minutes, 10 incline, 3.0 speed
2 minutes, 5 incline, 3.5 speed
Put the incline to 0
For the next 4 minutes, do the following -
30 seconds sprint
30 seconds rest
Repeat sprinting cycle 3 more times
Go to the elliptical and go at a good pace for 8 minutes
Finish on the stairmill and go at a good pace for 8 minutes

No Machines 1

2 sets:
-50 jumping jacks
-50 toe taps
-50 body weight squats
-50 calf raises
-50 total alternating lunges
-50 one legged deadlifts
-50 mountain climbers
-50 total step ups, alternating

No Machines 2

50 jumping jacks
10 push ups
10 burpees
50 pop squats
100 mountain climbers
1 minute air jump rope
Repeat 2 more times
Finish with a jog for about 5 minutes. No need to time - just estimate.

No Machines 3

Tabata time!
Do the following exercises for 20 seconds, and rest in between each exercise for 10 seconds.
-alternating lunges
-pop squats
-mountain climbers
-jumping jacks
-leap frogs
-jump lunges
-jog in place
-burpees
Rest for 1 minute
Repeat cycle 3 more times

No Machines 4

FINAL CHALLENGE!
Start with a light jog for about 5 minutes
10 push ups
20 side to side jumps
30 skaters
40 pop squats
50 crunches
60 jumping jacks
70 mountain climbers
80 alternating lunges (total)
90 high knee jog
100 squats
Finish with burpees to failure

Part Three – Other Ideas

I always tell people that a gym is great, but you don't NEED one to be healthy and fit. Here are some other ideas for exercise. You may hate the gym, can't make it one day, can't afford it, or just want something different to do for a workout. Whatever the reason may be, here are some ideas for you to try.

Go Outside
The possibilities are limitless. You can talk a walk by yourself or do one of the "no-machine" cardio routines I included in this book. Or call up a friend and enjoy a nice walk. Mix it up and have fun!

Join a Class
There are many options available for this. If you do have a gym membership, there may be classes offered for no extra charge beyond your monthly dues. If you don't have one, don't worry! There are other facilities that offer classes, anywhere from CrossFit, to hot yoga and Zumba. If you have a limited budget, go online and visit Groupon. Depending on your area, there may be hundreds of options for you at a very reasonable cost. Be daring and who knows if you will find something that you really love.

Hire a Personal Trainer

This may put some "spice" back into your workouts. Some gyms may even offer some free sessions. They tend to be on the expensive side. However, if you are able to hire one on a consistent basis, it could help with your goals. You will know that you need to meet with them on X date, so you may work a little bit harder.

Share a Trainer

Maybe you like the idea of a personal trainer, but you cannot afford it. Find out if you can share the hour with a few friends in a group session. Believe me, you will still get a good workout and it will be a lot of fun!

Find a Gym Buddy

I'm sure there are people at your gym that may in your same situation. Working out with someone else with similar goals can be encouraging and a lot of fun. Talk to people at the gym or find someone on social media to meet up with. You'll be able to push each other and reach goals even faster.

Non-Workout Ideas

So after reading this, you may feel like you mix up your cardio pretty well. However, maybe you're still bored and need something fresh. There are several different things that you can do to make you look forward to the gym and your next cardio workout. These include -

It is essential that you find a type of exercise that

you enjoy. It's definitely not mandatory to join a gym and do cardio as part of your routine. If the thought of getting on a cardio machine or even going to a gym makes you want to throw up, then don't do it. The point is just to exercise for health. There are numerous other ways to be active, and you should definitely find something that you enjoy and makes you happy.

New music - It is time to change up your music if you are able to know what song is coming up next. Just by changing your music, you may look forward to your next workout.

2. **YouTube -** do you have free wi-fi at the gym or sufficient data to watch videos? Make sure to still keep up the intensity, but there are hundreds of thousands of hours on so many topics on there to watch.

3. **New outfit, shoes or bag**

4. **Yummy healthy meal afterwards you can look forward to -** I used to make healthy protein ice cream, and it would "make" while I was at the gym. When a routine was tough, I'd think about my "ice cream" and it seemed easier.

Thank You!

I want to say THANK YOU for reading my book! I hope it helped you in your workouts and received some great value.

If you have any questions or comments, feel free to email me anytime at kelliraefit@gmail.com. I love receiving feedback and if you have a success story, share those too!

You can also follow me on Instagram @kelliraefit.

You May Also Enjoy

[42 Vegan Protein Shakes and Smoothies: Quick, Easy and Perfect For Clean Eating](#)

Made in United States
Orlando, FL
10 August 2023